Selina Eder

Palliative care for homeless people

Selina Eder

Palliative care for homeless people

Experiences, perceptions and wishes of homeless people and caregivers

ScienciaScripts

Imprint

Cover image: www.ingimage.com

This book is a translation from the original published under ISBN 978-620-0-44970-2.

Publisher:
Sciencia Scripts
is a trademark of
Dodo Books Indian Ocean Ltd. and OmniScriptum S.R.L publishing group

120 High Road, East Finchley, London, N2 9ED, United Kingdom
Str. Armeneasca 28/1, office 1, Chisinau MD-2012, Republic of Moldova, Europe
Printed at: see last page
ISBN: 978-620-8-28240-0

Contents

Summary

Background: People affected by homelessness often suffer from advanced, incurable illnesses and require palliative care. However, they are often denied access to this care for various reasons. The aim of this thesis is to present the perceptions, wishes and experiences of palliative care from the perspective of the carers and the homeless people themselves in a single work.

Research question: What are the experiences, perceptions and wishes of homeless people about their palliative care and how do carers view it?

Methods: A structured literature search was conducted in the Pubmed and CINAHL databases, as well as a hand search on Google Scholar, from October 2023 to February 2024. The titles, abstracts and full texts of the studies were then analysed using the previously defined inclusion and exclusion criteria, which were created using the SPIDER tool. Using Behrens and Langer's evaluation form, the previously identified four studies were assessed for quality and included in this paper.

Result: From 128 results of the structured literature search, four qualitative studies were included in this literature review to answer the research question. Thomas and Harden's guidelines for thematic analysis were used to compile suitable thematic groups. Five main themes emerged from this analysis: Place of dying, access to palliative care and care facilities, challenges in caring for homeless palliative care patients, homeless people's fears and wishes regarding their palliative care and coping strategies.

Conclusion: Access to palliative care for homeless people is limited. Increased presence of health services in hostels, training of staff in homeless shelters and greater multidisciplinary collaboration are needed to improve palliative care for this population.

Keywords: carers, homeless people, palliative care, perceptions

CHAPTER 1

1. Introduction

Firstly, the theoretical background of the research topic is explained in more detail. Then the problem situation, the nursing relevance, the research gap and the aim of this work are discussed.

1.1 Palliative care

Around 80,000 people die in Austria every year. Of these 80,000 people, 16,000 require specialised hospice or palliative care (Hospiz Osterreich, 2015). Palliative care is made up of palliative medicine and palliative care. While palliative medicine focusses almost exclusively on the medical aspects of care, palliative care focuses on the nursing care and other needs of patients. The aim is not to cure patients (Rosenberg, 2016), but to improve the quality of life of patients and their families when they are confronted with the challenges of a terminal illness (WHO, 2002). However, palliative care is not only provided to patients with a serious illness, but also to people who have reached the end of their lives as a result of an accident, for example (Rosenberg, 2016).

Another focus of palliative care is to recognise and alleviate pain and other physical complaints early enough (WHO, 2002). A combination of different analgesics can be used for this purpose. Palliative care can also take the form of therapies. An example of this is palliative chemotherapy. This is a form of treatment where the patient is administered cytostatic drugs that are not intended to cure a carcinoma, but to reduce pain and other physical discomfort. Another possible positive effect is that the administration of palliative chemotherapy can delay the growth of tumours (Rosenberg, 2016).

Other symptoms that patients may experience, such as breathing problems or nausea, are included in palliative care and alleviated or, in the best case, prevented altogether. This symptom control in turn aims to improve the quality of life (Rosenberg, 2016). Psychological and spiritual support are also integrated into palliative care (WHO, 2002). The aim here is to prevent or stop depressive moods, anxiety and emotional distress. Through this and other support, the aim is to enable patients to live comfortably, without pain and fear, until death (Rosenberg, 2016). However, the palliative care approach not only offers support to patients, but also to their relatives. However, this approach neither hastens nor delays death (WHO, 2002). It is about improving the remaining time (Rosenberg, 2016) and recognising that dying is a natural course of life (WHO, 2002).

1.2 Homelessness

Within the European Union, the number of homeless people has increased significantly over the last ten years (European Commission, n.d.). In 2021, the number of registered homeless people in Austria was 19,450, the lowest number since 2011. Since 2017, the number of registered homeless people has continued to fall (Mohr, 2024).

A person is considered homeless if they are living on the street or in public places such as parks or under bridges that cannot be considered living space or accommodation. People who have no fixed abode and therefore stay in emergency shelters for a limited period of time are also considered homeless. However, homelessness should not be confused with homelessness. The term homeless refers to people who live in facilities where the length of stay is limited and therefore there is no possibility of living there permanently. Examples of this are women's refuges, transitional shelters, asylums and hostels (FEANTSA, 2005).

1.3 Problem situation

Homelessness is one of the most radical forms of social isolation and has a significant impact on people's physical and mental health and well-being (European Commission, n.d.). In addition, homelessness leads to early death and thus increases the mortality rate. Looking at the average life expectancy of homeless people, it is 47 years, whereas homeless women only live to 43 (Bethan, 2012). In comparison, the average life expectancy in Austria is 78.3 years for men and 83.3 years for women (Statistik Austria, 2023). More recent data on the life expectancy of homeless people is not available. To ensure comparability, the data from 2012 was therefore also used for the average life expectancy of the Austrian population.

One reason why homeless people have such a low life expectancy is co-morbidity. Homeless people in the UK have a wide range of mental and physical illnesses. These include respiratory, gastrointestinal, joint and muscle diseases. There are also problems with the eyes or teething. Depression is very common among homeless people. More than one in three homeless people in the UK suffer from it (Homeless link, 2014). Other problems such as inadequate

Nutrition, personal hygiene and sleep problems are also very common among people experiencing homelessness. This is compounded by problematic access to healthcare and generally limited adherence to treatment, which have an additional negative impact on the health of the homeless population (Bethan, 2012).

Homeless people suffer more frequently from physical illnesses than the general population. In particular, eye problems, respiratory problems and problems with joints and muscles are very common among homeless people. Only in the case of cardiological complaints is the general population more frequently affected than homeless

people. Mental illnesses also affect homeless people more than the general population. In terms of mental illness, depression is the most common mental illness among homeless people, accounting for 33%. The percentage distribution of depression in the general population, on the other hand, is only 3%. Other mental illnesses that are common among homeless people are personality disorders, schizophrenia and post-traumatic stress disorder (Homeless link, 2014). Another problem that is common among homeless people is addiction (EMCDDA, 2023). Addictions related to alcohol or drugs are particularly common. In the study by Homeless link (2014), 39% of homeless people surveyed stated that they take drugs or had a problem with drugs from which they were recovering. Cannabis is considered the most common drug among the homeless population, with a consumption rate of 64% of the participants surveyed. Other addictive substances that are consumed are prescription drugs, amphetamines and benzodiazepines. Heroin is also frequently used by homeless people. The consumption rate here is 27% among the homeless. A problem with alcohol is or has been experienced by 27% of the 10
homeless people who took part in this study. One in six homeless people stated that they consumed alcohol on a daily basis (Homeless link, 2014).

People who experience homelessness and also suffer from a mental illness are among the marginalised groups in society with many stigmas (EMCDDA, 2023). It is precisely these stigmas, discrimination and previous negative experiences with services from the healthcare system that lead to a loss of trust in other healthcare providers (Lamb et al. 2012) and also represent a major obstacle in terms of access to these service providers (EMCDDA, 2023).

1.4 Care relevance and research gap

Homeless people are also a part of society who may need palliative care services at the end of their lives. It is of particular importance that they are accepted in their way of life. Although some homeless people may struggle with addictions, the aim of palliative care is not to treat them, but rather to ensure that they are accepted with their addiction. Homeless people may experience negative emotions such as resentment towards healthcare facilities, which can lead them to avoid facilities such as hospices, even though they could provide relief from their symptoms. Another important aspect is the provision of palliative medication for symptom control, even if this may have a positive impact on an existing addiction (Gerhard, 2015).

The Code of Ethics for Nursing also emphasises the link between nursing care and respect for human rights. It also emphasises the right to dignity and respectful treatment to which all people are entitled.

The following is written in the Code of Ethics for Nursing:

"Inherent in care is respect for human rights, including cultural rights, the right to life and freedom of choice, the right to dignity and respectful treatment. Care respects age, colour, culture, cultural affiliation, disability or illness, gender, sexual orientation, nationality, politics, language, ethnicity, religious or spiritual beliefs, legal, economic or social status and is provided without discrimination based on these characteristics." (ICN, 2021).

It can therefore be deduced from the Code of Ethics that dying people and people with a terminal illness are entitled to die under dignified circumstances. Compassionate death is understood to mean the alleviation of symptoms such as shortness of breath, pain or nausea. Freedom of choice is also an important part of the code of ethics. This includes, among other things, self-control. Here, people at the end of their lives can have a say in the care and support process. This can alleviate physical symptoms such as anxiety caused by a loss of control, for example through unconsciousness. Another point of autonomy would be that their mobility is maintained for as long as possible (Office of the Bioethics Commission, 2015).

In order to improve palliative care for homeless people, it is necessary to better understand the living situation of homeless people. Their fears and concerns about their impending death also need to be explored in more detail. What concerns they still have that they may not have thought about to this extent before. But also wishes that preoccupy them at this stage of their lives (Webb et al., 2020). In addition, it is important to explore how homeless people currently perceive their palliative care and what experiences they have had so far (Shulman et al., 2018). Carers' perceptions of palliative care for homeless people are also important so that care provision can be further optimised. This can minimise the barriers to accessing palliative care for a particularly vulnerable population group (McNeil etal., 2012).

1.5 Objectives and research question

To the author's knowledge, there are few reviews of palliative care for homeless people. The description of the experiences, perceptions and wishes of homeless people about their palliative care from the perspective of the homeless people themselves and the carers who look after them is not shown in any work. The aim of this bachelor's thesis is to close this gap and to show the experiences, perceptions and wishes of homeless people about their palliative care and the carers' view of it in this thesis.

This leads to the following research question:

What are the experiences, perceptions and wishes of homeless

homeless people have of their palliative care and what is the carers' view of this?

CHAPTER 2

2. Methodology

This chapter describes the methodological procedure of the structured literature search, including the inclusion and exclusion criteria. The assessment tool by Behrens and Langer (2010) was used to check the quality of the studies. The literature selection process is explained and presented using the PRISMA statement according to Moher (2009). The presentation of the literature search serves to emphasise the comprehensibility of the results and increase their credibility (Booth et al., 2016).

2.1 Literature research

To answer the research question, a systematic literature search was conducted in the period from October 2023 to February 2024. At the beginning, a rough search was carried out on Google Scholar with the keywords "palliative care" and "homeless" to get an overview of the current research situation. Additional keywords were then added to the search string by reviewing numerous articles and studies. These terms are explained in more detail in section 2.3 Search strategy. The search string was then used to conduct a search in the appropriate nursing-relevant databases Pubmed and CINAHL, as well as another hand search on Google Scholar.

The keywords were formulated using the SPIDER tool by Cooke, Smith and Booth and result from the research question described above (Cooke et al., 2012).

S - Sample: Homeless patients and carers

PI - Phenomenon of Interest: Experiencing the palliative care of homeless people

D - Design: Interviews, observations, discussions

E - Evaluation: Experiences of homeless patients and carers regarding palliative care for homeless people

R - Research: qualitative research results such as phenomenological studies, descriptive qualitative studies, grounded theory, ethnography

2.2 Inclusion and exclusion criteria

In this chapter, the inclusion and exclusion criteria and the exact search strategy that was taken into account in the literature search in the aforementioned databases are explained in more detail.

Table 1 shows the inclusion and exclusion criteria that were defined for the structured literature search. The language of the studies was limited to German and English. A further inclusion criterion was to only include people who had completed nursing training. This includes nursing assistants, specialised nursing assistants and qualified nurses. Furthermore, homeless people living in unstable housing were also included in the group of people. In addition, the age of the study population was set at 18 years or older. As this study is concerned with recording perceptions and experiences, quantitative studies were excluded.

	Inclusion criteria	**Exclusion criteria**
Group of people	- Homeless people - Nursing staff (PA, PFA, DGKP)	- People in stable housing conditions - Other professions from the healthcare sector
Age group	- >18years	- <18years
Research design	Qualitative primary studies such as - Grounded Theory	Quantitative Primary studies such as

	- Phenomenological Studies - Descriptive qualitative studies - Interviews	- RCT'S - CCT's - Cohort studies
Language	- German and English	- All other languages

Table 1: Inclusion and exclusion criteria

2.3 Search strategy

Suitable keywords were defined so that all relevant study articles could be identified in the two databases mentioned above. The keywords were: nurse, homeless person, palliative care and qualitative. In order to filter out all studies of qualitative research, the keyword qualitative was replaced by keywords of qualitative research such as wish, perception, fear, sorrow. This can be seen in the search string and in Table 2 Keywords and synonyms. Additional synonyms were added to the search string to increase the number of hits from the studies. The keywords are shown in the following table.

Keywords	**Plural**	**Synonyms**
nurse	Nurses	nursing
Homeless person	Homeless persons	homelessness
Qualitative	Desire, wish, request, fear, anxiety, trouble, sorrow, care, problem, perception, sense, cognation, percipience, awareness	Desires, wishes, requests, fears, anxieties, troubles, sorrows, cares, problems, perceptions, senses, cognations, percipiences,

		awarenesses
Palliative care		Terminal care, end of life care

Table 2: Key words and synonyms

Finally, the keywords are linked with the Boolean operators "OR" and "AND". In addition, truncations (*) are set in a database to include all word endings in the search. This resulted in the following search string for Pubmed:

(nurs*) AND ("homeless persons" OR homelessness) AND (desire* OR wish* OR request* OR fear* OR anxiety OR anxieties OR trouble* OR sorrow* OR care* OR problem* OR perception OR sense* OR cognation* OR percipience* OR awareness*) AND ("palliative care" OR "terminal care" OR "end of life care")

This search string was used for CINAHL:

nurse OR nurses OR nursing AND homeless persons OR homelessness AND desire OR desires OR wish OR wishes OR requests OR fear OR fears OR anxiety OR anxieties OR trouble OR troubles OR sorrow OR sorrows OR care OR cares OR problem OR problems OR perception OR perceptions OR sense OR senses OR cognation OR cognitions OR percipience OR percipiences OR awareness OR awarenesses AND palliative care OR terminal care or end of life care

A total of 127 results were obtained in the Pubmed and CINAHL databases. Pubmed accounted for 72 results and CINAHL for 55 results. In addition, a hand search was carried out in Google Scholar, where one further result was found. In addition, suitable reference lists were examined, but no further results were found. This research process was thus able to identify 128 results. After the duplicates (18) were removed, 110 publications were left for further research. These were then screened for relevance using title and abstract screening. This process identified 15 potentially relevant publications, which were subjected to full-text screening. As a result, eleven publications were excluded due to the previously defined exclusion criteria. This left four qualitative primary studies that met the defined inclusion criteria to answer the research question.

Some of the studies included in this work involve different occupational groups. Nevertheless, the focus of this thesis is exclusively on the perspective of carers and homeless people. Therefore, in studies with different perspectives, only the views of carers and homeless people were included in the results. If the results could not be clearly assigned to one occupational group, they were excluded. The four studies included in this paper were critically evaluated using the Behrens and Langer (2010) evaluation form. A PRISMA flow chart was used to visualise the study selection. This is shown in the following figure.

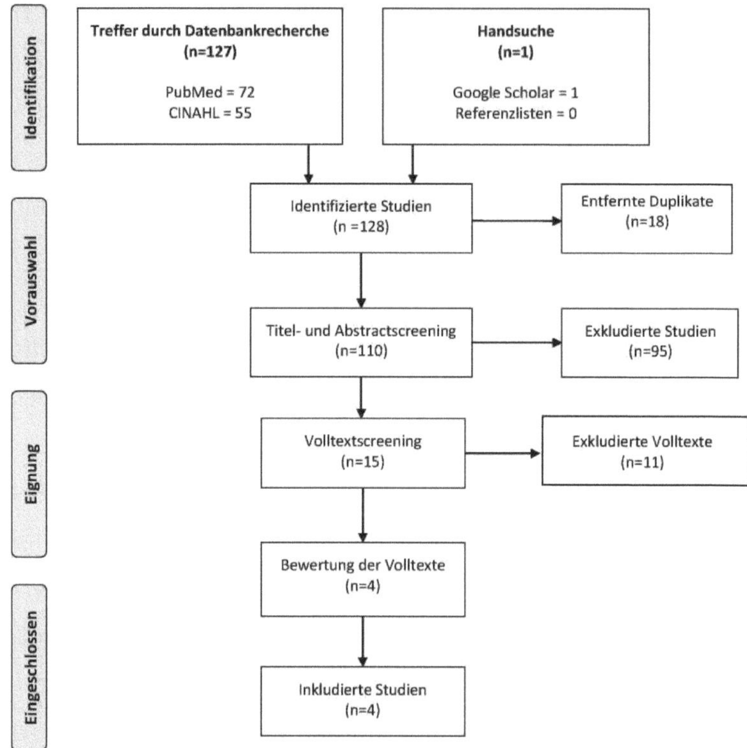

Figure 1: PRISMA Flow Chart 2009 (Moher et al. 2009)

Thomas and Harden's (2008) guidelines for thematic analysis were used to analyse the results of the studies and compile appropriate thematic groups. This process involved three steps: First, the full texts were searched for participant quotes and results to identify different thematic areas. Then, the statements and results identified were assigned to the previously defined topics. Finally, the themes and their content were compared, from which five descriptive thematic areas were derived (Thomas & Harden, 2008). These themes are as follows: Preferred place of dying, access to palliative care and care facilities, challenges in the care of homeless palliative patients, fears and wishes of homeless people regarding their palliative care and coping strategies.

2.5 Evaluation of the studies

The studies included in this bachelor's thesis were assessed for quality using the Behrens and Langer (2010) evaluation form. Based on the twelve questions contained in this evaluation form, the credibility, informative value and applicability were analysed. In addition, this assessment aims to evaluate the qualitative studies from a scientific perspective with regard to their objectivity and transparency (Behrens et al., 2022). The four studies included in this thesis were subjected to a critical evaluation. A detailed description of their quality and goodness can be found in the discussion section. The evaluation form by Behrens and Langer (2010) can be found in the appendix.

CHAPTER 3

3. Results

This chapter presents the results of the included studies. To this end, the study characteristics are presented graphically at the beginning in Table 3. This provides a structured and clear presentation of the substantive information. The table is organised as follows: Author, year of publication, country of publication, objective, setting and sample, method and results.

3.1 Study characteristics

Author:inside; Publication year and country	Title	Objective	Settingand Sample	Method	Results
Shulman Caroline, Hudson Briony F., Low Joseph, Hewett Nigel, Daley Julian, KennedyPeter , Davis Sarah, Brophy Niamh, Howard Diana, Vivat Bella, Stone Patrick (2018) United Kingdom	End-of-life care forhomeless people: A qualitative analysis exploring the challenges to accessand provisionof palliative care	This study examined the perspectives and Experiences from Homeless people, employees of the Aid for the homelessand Healthcare providers n with regard to Support for homeless people with advanced Disease and developed proposals for the Improvement of the Supply.	Sample: homeless people (n=28), formerly homeless people (n=10), health and social services social services (n=48), employees of emergency sleeping centres (n=30) and social workers (n=10). All participants are homeless or work with Homeless people in one of the three London boroughs	Design: more qualitative Research approach Data collection: semi-structured individual interviews and focus groups	This study emphasises that many homeless people die in unacceptable circumstances, which is a growing concern. It highlights the challenges of identifying palliative care patients and the lack of adequate care facilities for the homeless, especially for simultaneous drug abuse.

Authors; Publication year and country	Title	Objective	Settingand Sample	Method	Results
			together.		
De Veer Anke J E, StringerBarbara , Van Meijel Berne, VerkaikRenate , Francke Anneke L (2018) The Netherlands	Accessto palliative care for homeless people: complex lives, complex care	The aim of this study was to provide an insight into the extent to which people experiencing homelessness have access to good palliative care.	Sample: Homeless people (n=7), social workers (n=13), doctors (n=12), nurses (n=16), cares assistants (n=3) and a coordinator (n=3). assisted living (n=1) All Study participants are themselves homeless, and	Design: qualitative research approachz Data collection: Individual interviews withopen Questions	The study shows that homeless people often have a delayed onset of palliative care due to various factors. The course of the disease is Moreover , due to several reasons, homeless people are unpredictable. Further need Homeless people one more comprehensive care with regard to pain and Symptom control and

Authors; Publication year and country	Title	Objective	Setting and Sample	Method	Results
			are at the end of their lives, or work directly with homeless people.		psychosocial and spiritual aspects.
Webb Wendy Ann, MitchellTheresa , SnellingPaul , Nyatanga Brian (2020) United Kingdom	Life's hard and then you die: the end-of-life priorities of people experiencing homelessness in the UK	The aim of this study was to analyse the Worries, fears, Preferences and Priorities of people experiencing homelessness in the UKam End of life.	Sample: homeless people (n=21) All of the study participants are homeless and attend various facilities. Homeless people.	Design: Phenomenology Data collection: semi-structured individual interviews with open Questions	The study showed that spiritual and practical concerns are of great importance to homeless people. In addition, homeless people are afraid of being forgotten and prefer to die suddenly in order to avoid needing care or their self-determination to

Authors; Publication year and country	Title	Objective	Settingand Sample	Method	Results
	services professionals	this population group.	(n=7) and personal carers (n=4) All study participants are professionals from the health and social services sector and are involved in the care of homeless people in one of the six Canadian cities.		the end-of-life care of homeless people. The participants in the study also Recommendations that could have the potential to minimise these obstacles.

Table 3: Study characteristics

3.2 Favourite place to die

Two of the included studies looked at the place where homeless people who need palliative care will spend the end of their lives. In the study by Webb et al. (2020), homeless people were asked which place they would prefer for end-of-life care. They revealed that it is not the location that is important, but the attitude of the carers towards them. The participants stated that they appreciate being treated with kindness and respect. Since it is often not easy for those affected to trust people, it was also an important point that they feel comfortable with the staff caring for them and that they are in a place where they do not feel judged. One participant listed the emergency shelter as her preferred place because she feels well looked after there (Webb, 2020).

"/ know it's a bit odd... but [I'd ratherbe here] at the [name of] hostel. Because you feel safe and secure here (Tina - homeless person) (Webb, 2020)."

In the study by Shulman et al. (2018), the study participants also talked about their favourite place to die. Here, homeless people stated that the emergency shelter was their "home". So if that is where they wish to die, it should be made possible. They felt that it was the place where their emotional needs would be best met, even if a hospital could better take care of their physical needs. However, many saw hospitals as a "place of death". A visitor to the day centre recounts a conversation with a sick homeless man (Shulman etal. 2018):

"I remember one guy... his breath, you'd smell it, you'd know he was ill. And I used to say to him, get help ... get to hospital ...he just was absolutely terrified ofhospitals. He'd say 'hflc/o into hospital, I'm coming out in a box' (Day centre user - Borough B) (Shulman etal., 2018)."

3.3 Access to palliative care and care facilities

Another problem with access to palliative care is that the focus is shifting away from recovery. Recovery is not possible for everyone, so the focus is on living well until death. In London, there are homeless hostels where support services are offered to help people transition to alternative accommodation or to stabilisation and employment. It is difficult for the staff working there to recognise that recovery is no longer possible. However, if a homeless person requires more support due to an advanced illness, it is difficult to find a place in a care home. They do not fulfil the criteria for a place in a care home, often due to their young age. Added to this are possible behaviours associated with substance abuse, which presents a further challenge for care homes and hospices. For this reason, it is essential for this population group to utilise these services. One graduate nurse described it as follows (Shulman et al., 2018):

*"Most care homes are with people with dementia who are older; it's just, it's ourpatientsjust don't fit any of these like rigid things ... the care homes themselves are like 'what?! '*We *don't want this 29year old'... you know? (Specialist nurse - Borough C) (Shulman etal., 2018)."*

Another problem perceived by a carer in the study by de Veer et al. (2018) is that healthcare facilities are ambivalent about caring for homeless patients or are sometimes even reluctant to do so. For example, facilities often have difficulties dealing with the lifestyle of homeless people, as this group of people is generally unwilling to change their habits, for example to give up drugs. Furthermore, a qualified nurse stated that professionals in homeless facilities do not know the difference between palliative care and end-of-life care. For example, staff did not recognise that some patients need palliative care even though they are not in the final phase of their lives. However, one of the strengths of the staff in the homeless centres is to provide a safe environment for the residents there and to create a trusting relationship with the people there (De Veer et al., 2018). Another carer considers it important that all health and social care facilities, such as soup kitchens or emergency shelters, that are used by homeless people should work together. The staff at these organisations are in constant contact with this population group, so they would notice changes in their state of health and could then arrange access to the necessary healthcare providers. In addition, they have already built up the necessary trust with those affected and can therefore provide them with the best possible support (McNeil et al., 2012).

3.4 Challenges in the care of homeless palliative patients

In all included studies, challenges in the care of homeless palliative care patients were mentioned. Homeless study participants mentioned that they focus on the basic needs of daily life and live in what is known as "survival mode". This means living one day at a time (Webb et al., 2020). This is why they also find it difficult to talk about future preferences regarding the care they would like to receive. The following quote from a homeless person expresses this (Shulman et al., 2018):

A lot ofpeople are frightened to think about it. Most people won't talk about it, they won't entertain talking about it. They see it as so faraway, you know? Why bothernow, let's wait until nearer the time (Hostel resident - Borough C) (Shulman et al., 2018).

It is also not easy for care staff to talk to homeless people about their preferences regarding care needs. They fear that it could take away hope or give them a false sense of security if they broach the subject. There is also a concern that discussing their future health will negatively impact their emotional wellbeing (Shulman et al., 2018). Homeless people justified their refusal to have such a conversation because it would bring back painful memories. Therefore, being there for the sick person was seen as the most important thing (De Veer et al., 2018).

Another challenge in the care of homeless palliative care patients is that they find it difficult to trust other people and therefore inherently distrust the motives of others (Webb et al., 2020). Due to stigmatisation, denigration by professionals and the feeling of not being treated equally, there is a lack of trust in professionals in particular. As homeless people generally do not accept support easily, they find it even more difficult to ask for help due to the reasons mentioned. In addition, homeless people are also very concerned about maintaining their autonomy, which is diminished if they ask for help or accept it. One study participant from the care sector also describes how difficult it is to motivate homeless people to accept medical help, such as an annual somatic screening (De Veer et al., 2018). However, the problem is not only accepting help, but often also finding help that this population group can accept. People in care perceived that end of life care providers have introduced policies, such as the anti-drug policy, that deliberately deny homeless people access to these services. They also noted that homeless people who use drugs were categorised as disruptive by the person working at the reception of the end of life care facilities and were therefore excluded from care there. This was perceived as discriminatory by the carers who took part in the study by McNeil et al. (2012). This prevented this population group from accessing services and at the same time increased inequitable access to the end of life care system (McNeil et al., 2012).

One carer describes this in the following comment:

It's driven by the fact that the health care system has failed that population... When they are trying to access care in the mainstream facility, they experience discrimination and disrespect and poor care (Nurse) (McNeil et al., 2012).

Even with homeless people who have cancer, it is difficult to get a place in a hospice. Carers note that even if the homeless person does not take drugs, it is a challenge to get a place in a nursing home or hospice due to the usually young age of the person concerned and the unpredictable course of the disease. One carer describes (Shulman et al., 2018):

The last time I tried to get a [homeless] patient a bed at a hospice, they [the hospice] interrogated me. They wanted a very clear prognosis and it was because the woman I had sent there before, who we thought was dying ... was there formonths because she had nowhere else to go (Hospital palliative care nurse specialist - Borough B) (Shulman et al., 2018).

The course of a homeless person's illness is also difficult to predict, as a move from the streets to a flat, for example, helps to stabilise their state of health. This results in an unexpected temporary improvement for those affected. This is not only due to the move, but also to the care that these people receive there. Those affected are supported in adhering to medical treatments, suddenly have a change in food intake, a regular day-night rhythm and receive attention from other people. As a result, the person's health improves more quickly than would have been expected if they had remained in their previous environment. Care staff notice that as soon as the health condition improves, homeless people tend to return to their usual way of life and familiar surroundings as quickly as possible. This makes it difficult for staff to gain a good insight into the course of the disease, but emphasises the strong will to live of those affected (De Veer et al., 2018).

(John's nurse): "...we thought...this will not last long. But one way or another, he recovered again. He was admitted to hospital and we thought this is the end. But then...suddenly...aftertwo days he returned and was on the streets to take his heroin. As if he rose from the dead... I'll never forget his will to live (De Veer et al., 2018)."

The strong urge to use addictive substances is another problem in care that is difficult for professionals to deal with. Those affected spend a lot of time obtaining and consuming addictive substances such as alcohol or drugs. Accordingly, the social contacts of this population group are only based on people who also consume addictive substances. This instrumental behaviour makes communication with healthcare staff challenging and prevents genuine social contact. However, communication can also be limited for other reasons. Intellectual impairments, acquired through years of dependency or congenital, as well as psychiatric illness such as psychosis, can also restrict communication. This jeopardises the continuity of care and the relationship with professionals who go to great lengths to provide care and remind people of medical appointments or accompany them to hospital. When professionals were asked how they describe the difficult behaviour of homeless people, the following terms were used: aggressive, dismissive, passive, manipulative, norm and rule violating (De Veer et al., 2018).

People experiencing homelessness usually do not have any real social contacts. Their social network consists of other homeless people with whom they consume various addictive substances. When they fall ill, this social network usually disappears. Family connections do not exist or are usually non-existent due to events described by those affected as painful. A homeless person talks about the connection to his sister (De Veer et al., 2018):

"I have neglected herentire life. I only called herwhen I was in jail.
Then I ordered her to buy a game computer...that kind of things
(William, homeless) (De Veeretal., 2018)."

Psychosocial care was particularly difficult at the end of life. Carers noted that when the person was too ill to leave the room or spend time in a communal space, there was not enough time to go into the person's room and spend time with them, apart from the basic care provided and the serving of food. They also noted that some professionals did not realise that psychosocial and spiritual care are part of palliative care (De Veer et al., 2018).

3.5 Fears and wishes of the homeless regarding their palliative care

In the study by Webb et al. (2020), the homeless participants shared their experiences of palliative care. They also discussed how they would like to receive this care and what they are afraid of. In general, the participants did not think much about dying. However, almost all of them stated that they wished for a quick and painless death. Only one homeless person said that he wanted to know beforehand that he was going to die. When asked whether they would want medical help in the form of a lifesaving emergency, such as a cardiac arrest, more than half of the participants answered in the affirmative (Webb et al., 2020). Another major wish that is clearly recognisable in the study by Webb et al. (2020) is the maintenance of autonomy, which is very important to the participants. For example, most of the homeless people who took part in this study noted that they refuse medication that is used to treat anxiety, for example. The reason for this is that they do not want to lose control over themselves. For some participants, it also happened that their personal freedom was restricted because they were in a prison or psychiatric ward against their will. For this reason, it seems even more important to them to maintain control and preserve their autonomy (Webb et al., 2020). However, medication also poses a problem for another reason. If the homeless person is staying in a hostel or emergency shelter, the safe management of medication such as opioids is problematic. In addition, dying in a hostel or emergency shelter is an unpleasant experience for the other residents. One homeless person recounts this experience. It would be a disturbing factor if you had to walk past these people in the corridor. He describes the situation as follows (Shulman et al., 2018):

You've got to walk past those people [who are visibly unwell]. They half block the stairwell, you have to edge yourway past. It's kind of... in yourface. Erm, yeah, itbecomes part ofthe furniture. But it disturbs me as a person ... (Hostel resident- Borough C) (Shulman etal., 2018).

Because it is so important to the homeless to be independent and maintain their autonomy, the thought of becoming dependent and needing and accepting support is particularly difficult for them. This form of dependency is greatly feared by the homeless, even more than dying itself. The following quote underpins homeless people's fear of losing autonomy and the associated need for care (Webb et al., 2020).

'ending up in social care? That's my idea ofhell' (George - homeless person) (Webb et al., 2020)

Another fear of the homeless people interviewed in this study is being forgotten after death. They want other people to remember them and consider them important. Furthermore, some also expressed worries about where they will die and what will happen to them after their death. The fear of dying outdoors or in a place where they are alone unsettles the participants in the study. One homeless person stated that he had already seen many homeless people die outdoors and that the thought made him nervous. The so-called "burial of the poor" is also very popular among the homeless population. This refers to a burial that is financed from public funds. The cost of burial is generally a problem that burdens the homeless. The solution for a homeless person is (Webb et al., 2020):

'just put me on a fire ... and put the ashes on a council waste tip' (Justin - homeless person) (Webb et al., 2020)

3.6 Coping strategies

Faith and the power of God is a topic that is mentioned again and again by the participants. This topic helped many to get through difficult times. But humour and laughter were also mentioned by almost all study participants as a good coping strategy. One spiritual concern that many homeless people expressed was the issue of suffering. Therefore, especially in the study by Webb et al. (2020), many "Why me?" questions from the homeless in the interviews.

Wfty *do we all have to go through that suffering?' (Ray - homeless person) (Webb et al., 2020)*

CHAPTER 4

4. Discussion

The aim of this study is to highlight the experiences, perceptions and wishes of homeless people in relation to their palliative care and the care sector's view of this. Qualitative research was used to answer the research question posed above. Furthermore, the strengths and weaknesses of this work and recommendations for further research are discussed in this chapter.

Palliative care for homeless people is a very complex issue. There are many different experiences and wishes of homeless people with regard to their palliative care. The care perspective also brings with it some new perspectives. Despite the different views, the results of the included studies could be summarised in five categories. These are: "Preferred place of dying", "Access to palliative care and care facilities", "Challenges in the care of homeless palliative patients", "Fears and wishes of homeless people regarding their palliative care" and "Coping strategies".

The place of death is an important issue for homeless people. They want to die in a place where they feel comfortable and accepted. One person mentioned an emergency shelter as an example. (Webb et al., 2020). Hospitals, on the other hand, are terribly frightening for this population group, which is why they tend to avoid them (Shulman et al., 2018). Access to palliative care and care facilities is challenging for homeless people (Shulman et al., 2018; De Veer et al., 2018; McNeil et al., 2012). There is a lack of palliative care facilities, but also a lack of willingness on the part of care homes and hospices to accept these people and provide them with palliative care (Shulman et al., 2018; De Veer et al., 2018). Another challenge is the craving for addictive substances that many homeless people exhibit. This hinders communication with professionals and also leads to discriminatory behaviour towards them (De Veer et al., 2018; McNeil et al., 2012). The unpredictable course of the illness and the desire to return to their usual way of life as quickly as possible also hinders care (De Veer et al., 2018). It is particularly important for homeless people to lead a self-determined life. The need for care and the associated loss of autonomy, as well as the fear of being forgotten, are particularly feared (Webb et al., 2020). However, as homeless people live one day at a time, they also give little or no thought to future preferences in relation to their palliative care (Shulman et al., 2018).

Homeless people are afraid of becoming in need of care and thus losing their self-determination (Webb et al., 2020). They also have difficulties accessing care, just as care facilities have difficulties providing care for them. In addition, homeless people have often lost trust in professionals due to past trauma or feel that they are not treated equally or are stigmatised (De Veer et al., 2018). Research by Canavan et al. (2012) and Klop et al. (2018) shows that there are indeed prejudices against the homeless population in health services. Another study also shows that social services and care facilities are often unable to properly care for homeless patients with their multiple, complex problems (Schout et al., 2011). While hospitals are better able to meet the physical needs of dying homeless people, residential homes are better able to meet the emotional needs and have more experience in caring for people experiencing homelessness (Shulman et al., 2018). One reason for this is that general care homes and hospitals lack the skills to care for homeless people. However, shelters for homeless people lack expertise and palliative care options (Hudson et al., 2016).

The unpredictable course of illness of homeless people (Shulman et al., 2018; De Veer et al., 2018) due to a sudden change in their place of residence, for example by moving from the street to a flat, poses a further difficulty in determining the need for care. The move can cause a rapid change in health status and the associated need for care. It is therefore difficult to predict how care needs will develop (De Veer et al., 2018). Studies by Schanzer et al. (2007) confirm the significant improvement in health after a person moves into a sheltered environment (Schanzer et al., 2007).

4.1 Critical quality assessment of the included studies

The included studies are critically analysed in this chapter. Of the four studies included, one was rated as good, two as three and one as four. In general, some inadequate descriptions or explanations were identified, which will be critically analysed.

In the study by Shulman et al. (2018), there is no research question but two objectives that are clearly formulated. The participants were selected to match the research question. Former and current homeless people were recruited by the staff of the homeless shelters and day centres. On the negative side, there is no information in the study about how exactly the recruitment process took place or whether everyone who met the eligibility criteria was included. More transparency would be desirable here. Furthermore, the health and social care professionals were recruited via an existing professional connection to the research team. This means that the selection process is no longer objective. The exact number of study participants could not be determined either. The results section of the study mentions 127 participants, whereas the abstract mentions 126 participants. The absence of one person is never mentioned in the entire study. The data was collected using semi-structured interviews

and focus groups. However, the study does not mention the composition of these focus groups or how many participants per occupational group or population group took part in a focus group. For example, too many people per group led to too little speaking time, which could lead to a limitation in the number of participants.
The study does not refer to the perspectives represented. Likewise, the questions asked in the interviews are not mentioned in the study. Another shortcoming of this study is that it is not known whether or not data saturation was achieved after the ten semi-structured individual interviews and the 28 focus groups. It is therefore also not possible to say whether valuable information was lost or never picked up. On a positive note, the results were confirmed and there is a consensus within the research team. The results were also validated by the study participants.
The study by De Veer et al. (2018) was rated as good and only had minor shortcomings. On a positive note, the data collection was carried out up to data saturation. This was achieved after conducting 52 detailed interviews with people from different professions or population groups (homeless people, social workers, doctors, qualified nursing staff, care assistants, sheltered housing coordinators) about 19 cases of homelessness. Another positive factor is that the questions asked in the interviews are mentioned in the study. The recruitment of participants is also described in detail. The only criticism is that the contact person who approached the homeless people is not described. Furthermore, two of the researchers were briefly described and their experiences in qualitative research were also discussed. Another positive aspect of this study is that there was a consensus within the research team and validation took place in the form of two focus groups. It should be noted that the two focus groups each had

eleven participants. Of the eleven participants, ten were professionals and one was a representative of a homeless group. A better distribution of the participants would have been advantageous here in order to ensure precise validation of all previously made statements. Overall, the study has only minor shortcomings and the results of the study can be trusted.

The study by Webb et al. (2020) has one major flaw and several minor flaws. The participants in this study were selected according to the research question, but the result is not transferable to all homeless people in the United Kingdom, as the researchers imposed a language restriction. Only homeless people with sufficient knowledge of English were allowed to take part in the study. Another negative aspect of this study is that the exact questions used in the interviews are not mentioned in the study. There is only an interview schedule with four sections that was used as an interview guide. The topics of these four sections are known and are briefly mentioned in the study. Another criticism of this study is that there was no validation by the participants, nor is any information regarding consensus within the research team mentioned in the study. On a positive note, the data collection was carried out until a sufficient level of information and a high degree of meaningfulness was achieved.

The study by McNeil et al. (2012) has some shortcomings. For example, participants were identified according to the research question, but it was not mentioned how exactly they were identified. It is not known how exactly the identification took place and what criteria had to be met, other than that the person works in health and social care and is involved in the care of homeless people at the end of life. A more transparent procedure would have been desirable here. Another negative aspect to be mentioned is that no data was collected up to the point of saturation, which means that important impressions may not have been picked up. In addition, there was no validation by the study participants. On a positive note, an abridged version of the guidelines used for the interviews is presented in tabular form in the study. However, the exact interview questions are not mentioned. Furthermore, the data was analysed very carefully and attention was paid to the credibility of the categories formed. When revising the coding framework, attention was also always paid to consensus.

4.2 Limitations and strengths of this work

The strength of this bachelor's thesis can be seen in the broad-based literature search, which was carried out from October 2023 to February 2024. This research process was supplemented by a hand search and a search of the reference lists for suitable publications. In addition, the structure of this work is based on a systematic process. The formation of thematic groups according to the guidelines of Thomas and Harden (2008) can also be seen as a strength of this work. To ensure that the qualitative studies included in this review are credible, applicable and meaningful, their methodological quality was scrutinised. This was done using the Behrens and Langer (2010) evaluation form.

The evaluation of the studies can be seen as a limitation, as this was carried out by the author alone and relevant sources of error may have been overlooked. Furthermore, the linguistic restriction of the included studies to German- and English-language studies only represents a limitation. As a result, relevant studies in other languages may not have been taken into account.

Another limitation is that the healthcare systems from the countries in which the studies were conducted (United Kingdom, Canada, Netherlands) are not easily comparable with the Austrian healthcare system. As a result, the results are only transferable to the homeless population in Austria to a limited extent. Furthermore, during the selection process of the studies included in this thesis, some publications had to be excluded. The reason for this is that in some publications there was no clear distinction between homeless people, people in unstable housing and homeless people. As this thesis only focusses on homeless people, studies in which there was no clear definition of the study population had to be excluded from this bachelor thesis.

4.3 Recommendations for further research

Homeless people perceive their palliative care differently. The care sector also has different views on this topic. Homeless people are neglected in some areas or do not receive appropriate treatment. In addition, dealing with them is often difficult as their behaviour can be challenging. Nevertheless, they too have individual wishes, fears and needs that need to be explored and understood in order to improve their palliative care (Shulman et al., 2018; De Veer et al., 2018; Webb et al., 2020; McNeil et al., 2012).

In order to close the existing gaps in care, more research is needed to get an idea of the extent of the problem. Both a qualitative and a quantitative approach would be recommended. This would allow new proposals to close the gaps to be explored and then tested using a quantitative method.

It would also be necessary to carry out qualitative research in other countries to get a better overview of palliative care for homeless people in Europe. In addition, the results could then be better compared and the health systems could exchange information with each other in order to improve the palliative care situation for homeless people and facilitate access to health services for this population group. Above all, research in Austria is urgently needed, as no research on this topic has been carried out in Austria to date.

There is already evidence that interventions to require the preparation of patient summaries are an effective approach to meeting the needs of homeless people in their final phase of life. Nevertheless, further research is needed to verify the effectiveness of this intervention. It is also important to consider whether this intervention has been accepted by homeless people, as they are often less concerned about future preferences in relation to their palliative care and live more in the here and now.

4.4 Recommendations for practice

Based on the perceptions, experiences and wishes of homeless people and carers about palliative care for homeless people acquired through this review, significant recommendations for practice can be derived.

Homeless people have a reduced trust in the healthcare system and therefore often avoid healthcare facilities. For people who are or have been affected by homelessness, it is easy to make contact with other homeless people. Accordingly, care should be taken to ensure that homeless people tell each other about their palliative care needs. However, this is only possible if they share positive experiences, for example in hospital. This takes away the homeless people's fear and mistrust of the healthcare system and they are more willing to ask for help or admit that they need help and actively accept this help.

Another important point that needs to be improved in practice is the training of staff. Too little attention is paid to the challenging behaviour of homeless people and their special needs, especially during training. As a result, the negative attitude of staff towards homeless people is growing. It is important to learn how to deal with homeless people who require palliative care during training. However, it is not only dealing with the patients themselves, but also dealing with addictions in this context and the associated palliative medication that should be integrated into the training.

Discussions about future ideas of palliative care are rarely held, which can be attributed to various causes. To counteract this, these discussions should be held earlier in order to change the focus of the homeless person. In general, questions should not only be asked about the end of life. Rather, the focus should be on asking about wishes and decisions regarding the future. This will not only convey negative feelings to the homeless person and they may be more willing to talk about their preferences.

CHAPTER 5

5. Conclusion

Palliative care aims to improve the quality of life of patients and their families by alleviating suffering and recognising and treating pain and other physical and psychosocial problems at an early stage. However, it has been shown that homeless people have reduced access to this care. There are many reasons for this. On the one hand, society and healthcare facilities make it difficult for them to access it. In addition, they are repeatedly stigmatised and denigrated by the general public. On the other hand, it is a challenge to care for homeless palliative patients. They often lack trust in the healthcare system and are therefore reluctant to accept help. Dealing with this population group is made even more difficult by the unpredictable course of the disease. Their care needs can change rapidly due to a change in their location and lifestyle, which makes it difficult to plan ahead. In addition, their will to return to familiar environments and lifestyles as quickly as possible is not a requirement for care. Addictions are also common among homeless people and can have an additional negative impact on palliative care and make access to it more difficult. It is also difficult to enquire about their wishes in advance, as they give them little thought and usually do not want to give them up. They are too busy living one day at a time.

To summarise, palliative care for homeless people needs to be further improved to meet all their needs and give them equal access to palliative care services. This thesis aims to explore and better understand the experiences, perceptions and wishes of homeless people and carers in relation to palliative care for homeless people, in order to develop ways to further improve their palliative care.

Bibliography

Behrens, J., Langer, G. (2010). Evidence-based Nursing and Caring. http://www.medizin.uni-halle.de/index.php?id=572

Behrens, J., Langer, G. (2022). Evidence-based Nursing and Caring. Methods and ethics of nursing practice and health services research. (5th edition). Hogrefe. https://www.hogrefe.com/at/shop/evidence-based-nursing-and- caring-94218.html

Bethan, T. (2012). Homelessness kills: An analysis of the mortality of homeless people in early twenty-first century England. https://www.crisis.org.uk/media/236799/crisis_homelessness_kill s_es2012.pdf

Booth, A., Sutton, A. & Papaioannou, D. (2016). Systematic Approaches to a Successful Literature Review . InSAGE Publications (2nd ed.). SAGE Publications Ltd. https://www.researchgate.net/publication/235930866

Canavan, R., Barry, M. M., Matanov, A., Barros, H., Gabor, E., Greacen, T., Holcnerova, P., Kluge, U., Nicaise, P., Moskalewicz, J., Diaz-Olalla, J. M., Straftmayr, C., Schene, A. H., Soares, J., Gaddini, A., Priebe, S. (2012). Service provision and barriers to care for homeless people with mental health problems across 14 European capital cities, doi: 10.1186/1472-6963-12-222

Cooke, A., Smith, D" & Booth, A. (2012). Beyond PICO: The SPIDER tool for qualitative evidence synthesis. *Quality Health Research, 22*(10), 1435-1443. doi: 10.1177/1049732312452938

De Veer, A. J. E., Stringer, B., Van Meijel, B., Verkaik, R., Francke, A. L. (2018). Access to palliative care for homeless people: complex lives, complex care, doi: 10.1186/s12904-018-0368-3

European Commission. (n.d.). Homelessness. https://ec.europa.eu/social/main.jsp?catId=1061&langId=de

European Monitoring Centre for Drugs and Drug Addiction. (2023). Homelessness and drugs: health and social responses. https://www.emcdda.europa.eu/publications/mini-guides/homelessness-and-drugs-health-and-social-responses_en#section1

FEANTSA. (2005). ETHOS. European typology of homelessness, homelessness and precarious housing https://www.feantsa.org/download/at 6864666519241181714.

Pdf Gerhard, C. (2015). Praxiswissen Palliativmedizin: Konzept für unterschiedlichste palliative Versorgungssituationen(1st ed.). Thieme, https://doi.org/10.1055/b-002-101345

Office of the Bioethics Commission. (2015). Dying in death. Recommendations for the accompaniment and care of people at the end of life and related issues https://www.bundeskanzleramt.gv.at/themen/bioethikkommission/publikationen- bioethik.html

Homeless link. (2014). The Unhealthy State of Homelessness: Health audit results 2014. https://homelesslink-1b54.kxcdn.com/media/documents/The_unhealthy_state_of_homelessness_FINAL_1.pdf

Hospice Austria. (2015). Hospice and Palliative Care in Austria - Facts & Figures. https://www.parlament.gv.at/dokument/XXV/SNEK/670/imfname_381669.pdf

Hudson, B. F., Flemming, K., Shulman, C., Candy, B. (2016). Challenges to access and provision of palliative care for people who are homeless: a systematic review of qualitative research. doi:10.1186/s12904-016-0168-6

International Council of Nurses. (2021). The ICN Code of Ethics for

Nurses. https://oegkv.at/site/assets/files/10525/icn- ethik-kodex_broschuere_12-2021_fuer_web.pdf
Klop, H. T, Evenblij, K" Gootjes, J. R. G" De Veer, A. J. E" Onwuteaka-Philipsen, B. D. (2018). Care avoidance among homeless people and access to care: an interview study among spiritual caregivers, street pastors, homeless outreach workers and formerly homeless people, doi: 10.1186/s12889-018-5989-1
Lamb, J., Bower, P., Rogers, A. (2012). Access to mental health in primary care: a qualitative meta-synthesis of evidence from the experience of people from 'hard to reach[1] groups, doi: 10.1177/1363459311403945
McNeil, R., Guirguis-Younger, M., Dilley, L. (2012). Recommendations for improving the end-of-life care system for homeless populations: A qualitative study of the views of Canadian health and social services professionals, doi: 10.1186/1472-684X-11-14
Moher D, Liberati A, Tetzlaff J, Altman DG, The PRISMA Group (2009). Preferred Reporting Items for Systematic Reviews and MetaAnalyses: The PRISMA Statement. PLoS Med 6(7): e1000097. doi:10.1371/journal.pmed1000097
Mohr, M. (2024).Wohnungslose in Osterreich bis 2021. https://de.statista.com/statistik/daten/studie/958894/umfrage/woh nungslose-in-oesterreich/#:~:text=Wohnungslose%20in%20%C3%96sterreich %20bis%202021&text=Im%20Jahr%202021%20wurden%20in% 20%C3%96sterreich%2019.450%20Wohnungslose%20registriert t
Rosenberg, M. (2016). Palliative care: Quality of life at the end of life. Pflege.de. https://www.pflege.de/altenpflege/palliativpflege/
Schanzer, B., Dominguez, B., Shrout, P. E., Caton, C. L. M. (2007). Homelessness, health status and health care use.

doi:10.2105/AJPH.2005.076190

Schout, G., de Jong, G., Zeelen, J. Beyond care avoidance and care paralysis: theorising public mental health care. Sociology. (2011). doi:10.1177/0038038511406591

Shulman, C., Hudson, B. F., Low, J., Hewett, N., Daley, J., Kennedy, P., Davis, S., Brophy, N., Howard, D., Vivat, B., Stone, P. (2018). End-of-life care for homeless people: A qualitative analysis exploring the challenges to access and provision of palliative care. 36-45. doi: 10.1177/0269216317717101

Statistics Austria. (2023). https://www.wko.at/statistik/Extranet/Langzeit/Lang- Life expectancy.pdf

Thomas, J. & Harden, A. (2008). Methods for the thematic synthesis of qualitative research in systematic reviews. BMC Medical Research Methodology, 8(1). https://doi.org/10.1186/1471-2288- 8-45

Webb, W. A., Mitchell, T" Snelling, P" Nyatanga, B. (2020). Life's hard and then you die: the end-of-life priorities of people experiencing homelessness in the UK. 120-132. doi: 10.12968/ijpn.2020.26.3.120

World Health Organisation. (2002). WHO Definition of Palliative Care 2002. https://www.dgpalliativmedizin.de/images/stories/WHO_Definition_2002_Palliative_Care_english-german.pdf

Appendix

Critical assessment of a qualitative study

Source:

Research question:

Credibility

1. **Has the research question been clearly formulated?** Research topic discussed in its environment? Aims of the study defined?
2. **Which qualitative design was chosen and why?** e.g. ethnography, grounded theory, phenomenology
3. **Was a literature search carried out?** At what point in the investigation? Justification?
4. **Were the participants selected according to the research question and was the selection justified?** How was the selection made?
5. **Have the participants, their environment and the researchers been sufficiently described?** Also the perspective of the researcher?
6. **Was the data collection described in detail?** Method of data collection?
7. **How is the data analysed?** Codes, patterns, themes? Understanding hermeneutics
8. **Was the data collected up to the point of saturation?** If not, why not?

Significance

9. **Are the results detailed and comprehensible?** Process from data collection to topic development transparent? Quotes?
10. **Were the results confirmed?** Consensus in the research team? Validation by participants?

Applicability

11. Do the results of the study help me to better understand the people studied in their environment?

12. Are there concrete possibilities of application?

Credibility grading (bias avoidance): 1-2-3-4-5 - 6

http://www.medizin.uni-halle.de/index.php?id=572 V 1.1 from: Behrens, J., & Langer, G. (2010): Evidence-based Nursing and Caring. Hans Huber: Bern.

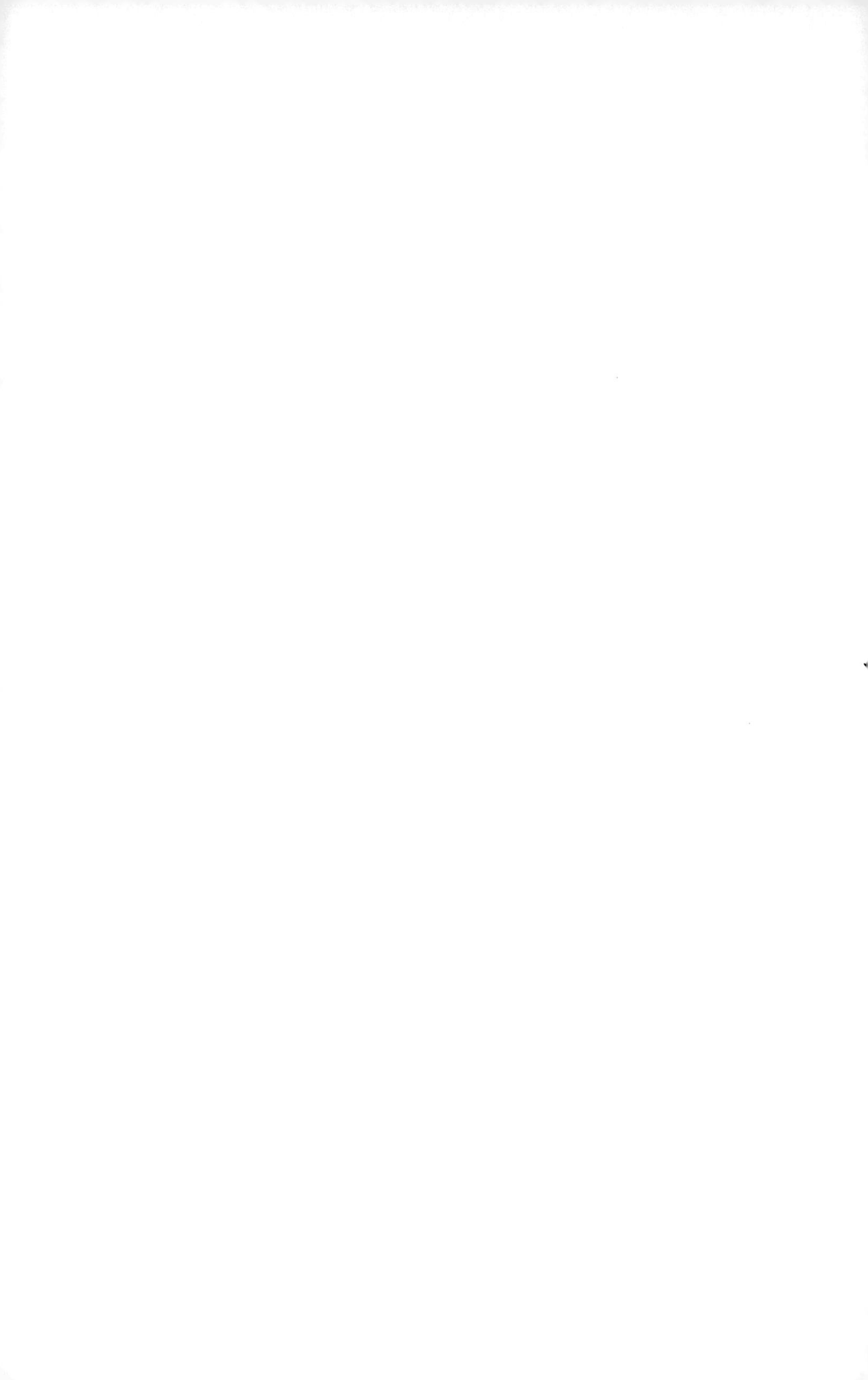

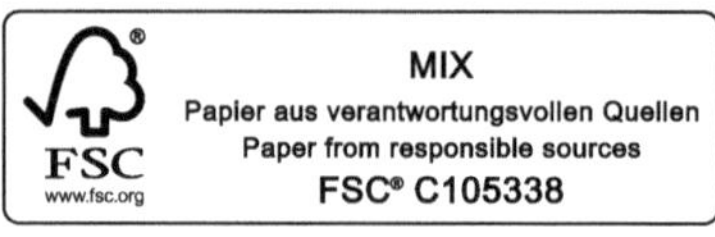

Printed by Books on Demand GmbH, Norderstedt / Germany